Book Of Salad Nutrition For A Great Health

Olatundun Solomon

olatundunsolomon@gmail.com

goodhealth1234567.blogspot. com

I have Honor Code Certificate from the University of Texas System edx. The course is 4.01x: Take Your Medicine-The Impact of Drug Development.

Am a Certified Alison Graduate with distinction in the course: Diploma in Nursing and Patient Care.

I have Honor Code Certificate from Harvard University through edx in the course PH201x: Health and Society.

Am a Certified Alison Graduate with distinction in the course: Diploma in Human Nutrition.

I also have Honor Code Certificate from edx Karolinska Institutet in the course KIBEHMEDx: Behavioral Medicine: A Key to Better Health.

It is very important to eat right, for the purpose of having a healthy body. The body needs enough nutrients to keep all the organs in the body in sound health. Malnutrition result to negative aspects to occur. For the body to be strong and vibrant proper care needs to be taken. The body needs salad in the diet. This helps to increase the immunity of the body. When the immunity of the body is increased, it helps the body to fight against any disease, therefore making the body to not be infected by the disease.

Salad as enough fibres that helps to

prevent colon cancer. Salad as

enough antioxidant that helps the

heart to function well. Salad as

enough vegetable oil that has

unsaturated fatty acid, this makes

fatty plaque not to be in the blood

vessels. This prevents

atherosclerosis. That is prevention of

fat accumulation on the inner wall of

the blood vessels that cause

narrowing of the blood vessels, that

result to high blood pressure. Salad

has enough fibres that helps to regulate the glucose level in the blood. Yellow fruits used as salad as beta carotene. This is good for a healthy sight of the eyes. This is because of the formation of vitamin A.

Folium in very green fruits is good for blood formation from the bone marrow. This prevent anemia (low blood level).

Salad

Salad is food that as combination of sliced vegetables or fruits, or with other food that are cooked for a healthy body.

Salad Recipe

Salad recipe is gotten from fruits, vegetables and cooked food. It is good to make all the recipe to be from a natural source. This prevent the risk of having cancer. Food that is synthetic, that has preservatives, colorants and additives are carcinogenic. Do not take alcohol.

Take non alcoholic drinks that are made from fruits. Alcohol can cause liver disease. This is very healthy for you.

Apple

Apple is a fruit that as fructose has sugar. This makes apple to be able to give enough energy to the body. It as enough fibres that makes colon cancer to be prevented. The green apple is good for blood formation from the bone marrow. Due to it's high fibre content it regulate the blood sugar. Therefore preventing hyperglycemia (too much glucose in the blood) and hypoglycemia (too little glucose in the blood). It is very good to eat the salad daily. Apple is good for proper brain function because of it's ability to give energy to the brain.

Apple Salad

Take healthy apples. That is apples

that are not infected by pathogens

(disease causing microorganisms).

 Wash the apples very well with

clean water.

Take a very sharp knife and slice the

apples into thin slices.

Put the slices into a plate.

You can eat it with a baked chicken

that has sliced onions, tomatoes and

spices inside. And also sprinkled

with small pinch of salt.

Too much salt can cause high blood

pressure.

The sliced onions inside helps to

prevent heart pain.

The sliced tomatoes inside the baked

chicken is good for a healthy sight,

because of the presence of beta

carotene. This makes vitamin A to be

formed in the body.

The spices inside the baked chicken

is good as antibiotics. This helps to

prevent infections to the body.

Banana

Banana is fruit that has enough vitamin K. It is good to prevent blood loss. When there is injury it stops hemorrhage(excess blood loss), by causing hemostasis (stop of blood loss).

Banana is sweet, it contain enough sugar that can give the body great energy.

Banana is also good to be eaten in order to prevent constipation (defecations does not occur).

It gives enough energy to the brain,

making the mind to function well.

Banana Salad

Take ripe bananas.

Use clean water to wash the

bananas.

Remove the banana covering.

Take a very sharp knife and wash

very well with clean water.

Cut the pilled bananas into slices.

Put the sliced bananas into a plate.

You can eat it with baked fish that as

spices and little pinch of salt

sprinkled on it.

Too much salt can cause high blood

pressure to occur.

Too much fried food can cause heart

problem.

Lemon

Lemon is a citrus fruit.

It has vitamin C.

It prevent scurvy. Scurvy cause

itching eyes and bleeding gums of

the mouth.

Lemon has enough fibre that

prevent colon cancer.

Lemon is acidic, it prevent infections

by pathogens.

It is good to treat fever.

Lemon Salad

Take lemon fruits and wash with clean water.

Take a very sharp knife and wash with clean water.

Remove the covering of the lemons with sharp knife.

Remove seeds of the lemons.

Slice the lemon into into slices.

Put the slices into a plate.

You can eat it with baked turkey that has slices of onions, tomatoes and chili in it. And having sprinkled salt on it. Too much salt can cause

hypertension (high blood pressure).

The tomatoes is good for eye vision

because of the presence of beta

carotene. That makes vitamin A to

be formed in the body. This prevent

myopia(short sightedness) and

hypermetropia(long sightedness).

The onions is good for proper heart

function and therefore, it prevent

heart pain.

The chili is spice, it act as antibiotic.

It prevent body infection by

microorganisms.

Green Beans

Green beans is protein food.

It has a lot of fibre that prevent

colon cancer.

It helps in the formation of blood

from the bone marrow.

It is good for healthy growth and development. It is good to replace worn out tissues. And it makes trauma(injury) to heal fast. This is because of the formation of new tissues.

Due to the formation of blood, it prevent anemia (low blood level).

Green Beans Salad

Take green beans and wash with
clean water.

Take a clean pot.

Put clean water into the pot.

Put the washed green beans into the
pot that is having clean water in it.

Cook until the green beans is soft.

Remove the green beans and put it
into a plate.

It is good to eat it with cooked rice
and tomatoes and pepper soup that
as fish in it.

The fish as oil that as omega 3 fatty acid. This is good for proper heart function.

The fish is protein, it helps for growth and development. It repairs worn out tissues.

The tomatoes as beta carotene that is good for a healthy sight.

The pepper is spice, it helps as an antibiotic. It is good to treat fever. It also prevent infection of the body by pathogens (disease causing microorganisms.

Corn Kennels

Corn kennels is carbohydrate.

It gives energy to the body.

It has a lot of fibre that prevent

colon cancer.

The yellow corn kennel has beta

carotene. This makes vitamin A to be

formed in the body. This is good for

healthy vision.

Corn Kennel Salad

Take corn kennels and wash with
clean water.

Take a clean pot.

Put clean water into it.

Put the washed corn kennels into it.

Put little pinch of salt into it. Too
much salt can cause hypertension
(high blood pressure).

Cook the corn kennels until it is soft.

Put the cooked corn kennels into a

plate.

It is good to eat it with cooked rice

and soup that as beef meat in it.

Rice gives energy.

Beef meat is protein. It helps for

growth and development. It also

helps for the formation of blood.

Tomatoes

Tomatoes is having beta carotene.

This is good for the formation of

vitamin A. This is good for healthy

vision.

It prevent colon cancer because it

has fibre.

It has a lot of fluid. This prevent

dehydration of the body. This makes

the blood to flow easily to all parts

of the body.

Tomato Salad

Take fresh tomatoes.

Wash the fresh tomatoes.

Take a sharp knife and wash it very

well.

Use the sharp knife to cut the

tomatoes into slices into a clean

plate.

You can eat it with sliced cabbage

that is washed.

And with cooked egg.

And also with baked fish that has

spices on it.

That cabbage helps in the immunity of the body.

It prevent colon cancer because of it's high fibre content.

The fish is protein. It helps in growth and development.

The egg is protein. It helps in the growth and development of the body.

The yolk of egg has beta carotene. This makes vitamin A to be formed in the body. This helps for a healthy vision.

The spices are good as antibiotics.

This helps to treat fever. It also

prevent infection of the body by

pathogens (disease causing

microorganisms).

Cucumber

Cucumber is a fruit that has high

fibre content. This makes it to

prevent colon cancer.

Cucumber as calcium, magnesium and potassium.

The calcium and magnesium helps for the formation of bone and teeth.

The potassium is good for heart and nerve health.

Green cucumber is good. It helps in the formation of blood.

Cucumber as high water content. This makes it to prevent dehydration of the body.

Very green cucumber when sliced and rubbed on the face, it prevent pimples and other skin infections.

Very green cucumber is good to treat fever. And also prevent diseases.

Cucumber Salad

Take cucumbers and wash with clean water.

Take a sharp knife and wash with clean water.

Use the sharp knife to cut the cucumbers into slices into a clean plate.

You can eat it with whole wheat bread and cooked egg that as spices on it.

The cooked egg is protein. It helps for growth and development. And also for the repair of worn out tissues. The yolk in the egg has beta carotene. This makes vitamin A to be formed in the body. This is good for good eye vision.

Spices is antibiotic. It treat fever. It prevent infections from bacteria and other disease causing microorganisms.

Whole wheat bread is good. It as fibre that is good to regulate the body glucose level. This helps to prevent hyperglycemia (too much sugar in the blood) and hypoglycemia (low sugar in the blood). Therefore diabetes mellitus(frequent urination that is having too much sugar in it) is prevented. Obesity is also prevented.

Carrot

Carrot is fruit that has beta carotene. It helps in the formation of vitamin A in the body. This helps in good vision. This prevent myopia (short sightedness) and hypermetropiav(long sightedness).

Carrot has a lot of fibre. This is good to prevent colon cancer and constipation (inability to defecate).

Carrot has liquid content. This helps to prevent dehydration of the body.

Carrot Salad

Carrot salad is prepared by taking carrots.

Wash them with clean water.

Take a sharp knife and wash it with

clean water.

Cut the carrots into thin slices into a

plate.

You can eat it with cooked rice soup

that has chicken and spices in it.

The rice is carbohydrate. It gives

energy to the body.

Unpolished rice has vitamin B. This

prevent beriberi.

The chicken is protein. It is good for

growth and development. It prevent

high cholesterol level in the body.

This prevent heart disease.

Spices are antibiotics. This helps to

prevent infections and treat fever.

Coconut

Coconut is a fruit that as oil. This oil

prevent heart pain.

Coconut as a lot of fibres, this

prevent colon cancer.

Coconut as liquid in it. This prevent

dehydration of the body.

Coconut Salad

Coconut salad is prepared by taking

a coconut.

Wash well with water.

Break the hard covering.

Remove the hard covering.

Wash the inner part that is having white part.

Take a knife and wash it with clean water.

Cut the washed coconut that is having white part into thin slices into a plate.

You can eat it with barbecued plantain. And washed sliced lettuce added to it.

The lettuce is good for the formation of blood. It has a lot of fibres that is good for prevention of colon cancer.

The plantain is carbohydrate. It gives

the body energy.

Pineapple

Pineapple is a fruit that has a lot of

fibre. This helps to prevent

constipation (inability for defecation

to occur).

It has vitamin K . This helps blood

clot to occur to an injury. Thereby,

preventing blood loss.

Pineapple has sugar in it. This makes it to give energy to the body.

Pineapple Salad

Take a ripe pineapple.

Wash it very well.

Take a sharp knife, and wash it very well.

Use the sharp knife to remove the outer part of the pineapple.

Cut the pineapple into thin slices, into a plate.

You can eat it with doughnut and fish that is cooked that is having spices on it.

The doughnut is carbohydrate. It gives energy.

Spices are antibiotics. This prevent infections and treat fever.

The oil in the fish as omega 3 fatty acid. The prevention of heart disease happens. It also prevent high blood pressure. It also prevent high cholesterol level in the body.

The fish is protein. It helps in the growth and development of the body.

Water Melon

Water melon has a lot of liquid. This helps to prevent dehydration.

It has sugar in it. This gives the body energy.

Water melon helps in the body immunity to be high. This helps to prevent diseases. The body is able to

fight against diseases.

Water Melon Salad

Water melon salad is prepared by

taking a ripe water melon fruit.

Wash it very well with water.

Take a sharp knife and wash it very

well.

Cut the water melon open. And

remove the outer part of it.

Remove the seeds.

Cut the soft part into small sections,

into a plate.

You can eat it with cake and cooked

beans that has fish, tomatoes and

pepper in it.

The cake gives energy.

The cooked beans is protein, it is

good for growth and development. It

helps to repair worn out tissues.

The tomatoes has beta carotene.

This helps in the formation of

vitamin A in the body. This helps in good vision of the eyes.

The pepper is spice. It is good as antibiotics. It prevent infection of the body by disease causing microorganisms. It treats fever.

Onion

Onion is vegetable. It has a lot of fibre. This prevent constipation (inability for defecation to occur).

It has potassium, calcium, fluoride, magnesium and vitamin C.

The magnesium and calcium helps the teeth and bones to be strong.

The fluoride prevent tooth decay.

The potassium helps the heart to function well. This prevent heart pain.

Due to it's high fibre, it prevent colon cancer.

It treat fever and prevent infection of the body by pathogens.

It is good to be used on the sight of the body that scorpion stung.

Onion is good to be used to prevent bad breath.

Onion Salad

Take onions and wash well with clean water.

Take a knife and wash well with clean water.

Cut the onions into small sizes, into a plate.

You can eat it with, roast meat that as pinch of salt and spices on it. And also with washed sliced cucumber.

The meat is protein. It helps for the growth and development of the body. It repair worn out tissues. It also helps for the production of blood from the bone marrow.

Use a little pinch of salt. Too much salt can cause hypertension(high blood pressure).

The cucumber as a lot of fibre. This helps to prevent constipation (the inability for defecation to occur). It also helps the immunity of the body. The body is able to fight against infections.

The spices helps as antibiotics. It treat fever. It prevent infections from happening to the body.

Soursop

Soursop is a fruit that is good to be eaten to prevent cancer.

It as a lot of fiber that makes

defecation to be possible.

It increase the body immunity

against infections.

Soursop Salad

Take a ripe soursop.

Wash it very well with water.

Take a sharp knife.

Wash the sharp knife with water.

Cut away the outer covering of the soursop fruit.

Cut the inner part of the soursop fruit into sections, into a clean plate.

You can eat it with cooked soup that as fish and beef in it. And eat it also with bread.

The beef and fish are protein.

The beef and fish helps for the growth and development of the body.

The fish has omega 3 fatty acid that

is good for good heart function.

The beef is good for the production

of blood.

The bread gives energy to the body.

Avocado

Avocado is a fruit that is good to

treat arthritis.

Avocado prevent arthritis.

Avocado helps to prevent joint

friction.

It prevent cartilage wearing.

It prevent bone wearing.

It prevent joint pain.

It increase body immunity. This
helps the body to fight against
diseases.

Avocado has a lot of vitamin K. This
helps in blood clot after injury.
Therefore preventing blood loss.

Avocado Salad

Avocado salad is prepared by washing it with water.

Take a sharp knife.

Wash the sharp knife with water.

Remove the outer covering with the clean knife.

Cut the soft part into sections, into a clean plate.

You can eat it with bread and tea.

The tea has theophyline which prevent heart pain.

The tea increase the body immunity.

This helps the body to fight against

infections.

The bread gives energy to the body.

This prevent fatigue (weak body).

The brain is able to function well.

The body as enough energy for

exercise. This makes the body to be

healthy.

Potato

Potato is carbohydrate.

It give energy to the body.

This makes the brain to have energy

to function well.

This makes the body to have energy

to be in normal condition.

Potato Salad

This is prepared by taking some

potatoes.

Wash the potatoes with clean water.

Take a knife.

Wash the knife with soap and water.

Take the clean knife to remove the outer part of the potatoes.

Cut the inner part of the potatoes into sections.

Put clean water into a pot.

Put the sections of the potatoes into the pot that has water in it.

Put little pinch of salt. Too much salt can cause hypertension(high blood pressure).

Cook until the potatoes is soft.

Put the cooked potatoes into a clean

plate.

You can eat it with baked fish that

has spices on it. And also with

sectioned lettuce and cucumber.

Cabbage

Cabbage is a vegetable.

It has vitamin C and vitamin K.

Vitamin C prevent scurvy (itching eyes and bleeding gums).

Vitamin K cause the blood to clot after an injury.

It gives the body high immunity.

It has a lot of fibre, this helps to prevent colon cancer.

It has a lot of fibre, this makes peristalsis to occur well in the intestine. This prevent constipation.

Cabbage makes the bone marrow to produce blood well. This makes anemia(low blood level) to be

prevented. This makes the body to

be well nourished.

Too much of cabbage consumption

can cause goitre (swollen thyroid

gland). This can be prevented by

putting iodized salt into food.

Cabbage Salad

Cabbage salad is prepared by taking

a cabbage.

Wash it very well with clean water.

Remove the layers one after the

other.

Cut into smaller sections, into a plate.

You can eat it with cooked rice,

sectioned clean carrots and soup

that has turkey in it.

Chili Pepper

Chili pepper has a lot of fibre, this

prevent colon cancer and

constipation.

Chili pepper is spice. This makes it to

be an antibiotic. It prevent infection

of disease and it treats fever.

It is good for good eye sight, because

it has beta carotene. This makes

vitamin A to be formed in the body.

Chili pepper also has vitamin C. This

makes scurvy(itching eyes and

bleeding gums) to be prevented.

Chili pepper should not be eaten

when there is stomach ulcer and

intestinal ulcer. Treatment of the

ulcer should be done in the hospital

by a medical doctor. After which chili can be eaten.

Chili Pepper Salad

Take chili peppers.

Wash the chili peppers with clean water.

Take a sharp knife.

Wash the sharp knife with soap and water.

Take the clean knife and cut the chili

peppers into sections, into a clean

plate.

You can eat it with barbecued meat

and sliced cucumber and cabbage.

The meat is protein. It helps for the

growth and development of the

body.

The meat also helps for the

formation of blood from the bone

marrow.

The cucumber has a lot of fibre that

helps to prevent colon cancer. It

prevent constipation. It also has a lot of fluid that hydrate the body when it is eaten, this prevent dehydration.

Cucumber also makes the body to produce blood from the bone marrow.

The cabbage has a lot of fibre it prevent constipation and it prevent colon cancer.

Cucumber increase the body immunity. This makes the body to be resistant against diseases.

Pawpaw

Pawpaw is a fruit.

It has a lot of fluid, this makes the body not to dehydrate.

It has sugar, this makes it to give energy to the body.

It has beta carotene, this makes vitamin A to be formed in the body. This is good for good eye sight.

Pawpaw prevent constipation (defecation inability).

Pawpaw Salad

Pawpaw salad is prepared by taking ripe pawpaw.

Wash it with clean water.

Take a sharp knife and wash with soap and water.

Take the clean knife and remove the outer layer of the pawpaw.

Cut the pawpaw open.

Remove the seeds.

Cut the pilled pawpaw into sections, into a clean plate.

You can eat it with toast bread and baked fish.

The bread gives energy to the body.

The fish is protein.

The fish cause growth and development in the body.

The fish helps in the repair of worn out tissues.

The fish has omega 3 fatty acid. This helps to prevent heart pain.

Lime

Lime is a fruit.

It is acidic.

It treats fever.

It has a lot of fibre. This makes it to prevent colon cancer. The fibre make peristalsis and segmentation to occur well. This prevent constipation.

It is acidic, this makes it to prevent infections. It also treat fever.

It is citrus fruit, it has vitamin C.

It prevent scurvy (itching of eyes and

the bleeding of gums in the mouth).

Lime Salad.

Lime salad is prepared by taking

some lime fruits.

Wash them with clean water.

Take a sharp knife and wash it with

soap and clean water.

Take the clean sharp knife to remove

the outer part of the lime.

Remove the seeds.

Cut the lime the outer part and

seeds are removed. Cut the

remaining parts into sections, into a

clean plate.

You can eat it with baked chicken

that as sliced onions and sliced

spices in it.

The chicken is protein. It helps for

body growth and development.

The onions is good to prevent heart

pain. It also as fibres this prevent

constipation and colon cancer.

The spices is antibiotic, it treats

fever and prevent disease infections.

Lettuce

Lettuce is vegetable.

It makes the bone marrow to

produce blood, this is because it has

iron and folium.This prevent anemia

(low blood level).

It has a lot of fibre, this prevent

constipation and colon cancer.

It increase the body immunity,

making the body to be able to fight

against diseases.

It has vitamin K. This makes clot of

blood to occur after injury.

It has vitamin A. This makes the eyes

to have normal sight.

Mango

This is fruit.

It has beta carotene. This makes

vitamin A to be formed in the body.

This helps for a good eye sight.

It has sugar, this provide energy to

the body.

It has fibres. This helps to prevent

colon cancer. And also prevent

constipation.

It has a lot of fluid. This makes it to

prevent dehydration of the body.

Mango Salad

Mango salad is prepared by taking
some mangoes.

Wash them well with water that is
clean.

Take a sharp knife and wash it with
soap and water.

Take the clean knife to cut the
mangoes and leave the seeds
separated.

Cut the parts that has been

separated from the seeds into

sections, into a clean plate.

You can eat it with sandwich and

honey.

The honey as sugar. This makes it to

give energy to the body.

The honey does not cause

hyperglycemia and diabetes mellitus.

The honey does not cause obesity. It

is also good to go for exercise for the

body to be healthy.

The sandwich provide energy and
other nutrients to the body. This
makes the body to be normal.

Ginger

Ginger is spice.

It as potassium, vitamin C,
magnesium and calcium.

The calcium and magnesium helps
for a healthy bone and teeth
formation.

Vitamin C helps to prevent scurvy (bleeding gums and itching eyes).

The potassium in ginger helps the heart to function normally.

Ginger is good for the heart to function normally.

Ginger has a lot of fibre, this prevent constipation and colon cancer.

Ginger prevent infections and treats fever.

Ginger has magnesium, this makes the bones of the body to be strong.

Ginger Salad

Ginger salad is prepared by taking ginger and wash it very well with clean water.

Take a sharp knife. Wash the sharp knife well with soap and water.

Cut the ginger into sections, into a plate.

You can eat it with baked fish, sliced cabbage and honey.

The honey give appetite and energy.

The fish is protein, this helps for
growth and development of the
body.

The fish has omega 3 fatty acid. This
helps to make the heart to function
well.

The sliced cabbage has fibres, this
prevent colon cancer and
constipation.

And the cabbage has vitamin C, this
prevent scurvy (itching eyes and
bleeding gums).

Cabbage also has vitamin K, this makes blood to clot after trauma (injury).

Garlic

Garlic is a vegetable.

It has phosphorus this makes the bones to be strong. The phosphorus helps in contributing to the structure of DNA(deoxyribonucleic acid) and RNA(ribonucleic acid).

Garlic as calcium and magnesium, these helps in the formation of healthy bones and teeth.

It has vitamin C this prevent scurvy (bleeding gums and itching eyes).

It has fibres this prevent constipation and colon cancer.

Garlic Salad

Garlic salad is prepared by taking garlic and wash it well with water.

Take a sharp knife and wash it with

soap and water.

Use the sharp knife to cut the garlic

into sections, into a clean plate.

You can eat it with baked fish and

roast meat that has spices on it. It is

good to add honey.

The fish and meat is protein. This is

good for growth and development of

the body. It repair worn out tissues.

The spices is antibiotics. This treats

fever and prevent infection of the

body from diseases.

The honey has sugar it gives energy to the body. It is also good as an appetizer.

Salad can also be prepared by mixing different fruits and vegetables that are sliced into a plate.

For example, take apples, carrots, cucumber, lettuce and cabbage.

Wash them all.

Use a clean sharp knife and slice

them into a clean plate.

Remove the seeds of the apple.

Eat them, this is highly nutritional.

You can also take other varieties of

fruits wash them very well with

water. And use a clean knife to slice

them into a clean plate.

You can eat it with honey and baked

chicken that has spices on it and

within it.

This is good for your body to be healthy.

It is good to eat natural food that has no preservatives, no additives and no colorants this prevent malnutrition and cancer. This makes the body as a whole to be healthy.

Guava Salad is good for a bleeding gums. And also for itching eyes, because of the presence of vitamin C(ascorbic acid). It is good to add unto it ginger drink. Ginger drink

helps to prevent heart diseases.

Guava salad can be prepared by

washing guava with clean water. Use

clean knife to cut the guava and

remove the seeds. Put it into a clean

plate.

The ginger drink can be prepared by

washing ginger, put it into a clean

blender machine. Blend it very

smooth. Put it into a clean jug. Add

clean water. You can add honey.

Steer well. Pour from the jug into a

cup. Eat the guava salad and drink
the ginger drink that has honey in it.
The ginger prevent heart disease.
The honey gives energy because it
has sugar. The guava prevent itching
of the eyes and bleeding gums
because it has ascorbic acid(vitamin
C). It is good to drink enough water
it prevent heart pain. It makes the
blood to flow easily to different
parts of the body.

Apple Salad and Baked Peanut

Apple salad and peanut is very good to be eaten for the under nourished. Those that are malnourished will regain to normalcy speedily. Apple has a lot of minerals that makes the body to be healthy. It is also good to drink milk because it has protein , vitamins and minerals. Soy milk is also good because it has vitamins and minerals. Cooked egg is also good to be eaten because it has a lot of nutrients. It makes the undernourished to be normal. It is also good to drink enough water in order not to be dehydrated.

Whole wheat bread, brown rice, cereals and vegetables is good to prevent anemia(low blood level).

The cereals is good source of vitamin B and green vegetables is good source for folium this helps in the production of blood from the bone marrow. This makes anemia to be prevented. When the body has enough blood, it makes the blood to nourish different parts of the body effectively. This prevent joint pain. This prevent diseases that is due to lack of blood supply.

Blackberry

Blackberry is very good. It is sweet, it gives energy. It makes somebody to have appetite to eat.

It is good for you to brush your mouth with fluoride toothpaste and toothbrush that is having small head and soft bristles. This prevent teeth discoloration and tooth decay. It

prevent teeth cavitation.

Cooked Yellow Corn And Coconut.

Cooked yellow corn has vitamin A

which is good for a healthy sight and

normal growth. Coconut has

unsaturated fatty acids which is

good for heart to function normally.

Garden Egg.

It is good to eat garden egg. It is good as disinfectant. It prevent infection of the mouth, intestines, skin and other parts of the body. It is good to treat fever. It is also good for the formation of blood from the bone marrow.

Strawberry Salad.

Strawberry is very good for the body. It as fluoride, this prevent tooth caries. It as calcium, magnesium and phosphorus that is good to make the bones to be strong. It had vitamin C.

Vitamin C helps to treat

scurvy(itching of the eyes and

bleeding gums). This prevent blood

loss that is due to bleeding gums.

This makes anemia to be prevented.

This makes soft bone(osteomalacia)

to be prevented. This makes

osteoporosis to be prevented. This

prevent bone fracture. This prevent

gum inflammation (gingivitis). This

prevent mouth infection. This

prevent the infection of other parts

of the body from mouth infection. It

is good the brush the teeth after eaten. It prevent mouth odour and mouth infections. Use fluoride toothpaste mouth odour will be prevented. This makes the mouth to be fresh and clean. This makes the mouth to have oral hygiene.

Kiwi Fruit Salad

Kiwi fruit has vitamin A. Vitamin A is good for a healthy sight.

It also has vitamin C this helps to treat scurvy (bleeding gums and itching eyes).

It has magnesium, calcium and phosphorus which helps to prevent weak bones. It makes the bones of the body to be strong.

Raspberry Salad

Raspberry salad is nutritious to the body. It has vitamin C, calcium, magnesium and phosphorus.

The vitamin C prevent itching eyes and bleeding gums. The magnesium, calcium and phosphorus helps the body to build a healthy bones and teeth.

The vitamin helps the body to have high immunity.

Pumpkin Salad

Pumpkin salad is very good to make the body healthy. It has vitamin A and vitamin C. Vitamin A makes somebody to see well. Vitamin C treats itching eyes and bleeding

gums.

Pumpkin also has vitamin K. Vitamin

K helps the body to stop bleeding

when there is injury. It cause blood

clot.

Pumpkin has calcium, magnesium

and phosphorus which makes the

bones to be strong.

Squash Salad

Squash salad brings good health to the body. It has vitamin A and vitamin C. Vitamin A is good for a healthy eye sight. Vitamin C is good to prevent bleeding gums and itching eyes. The vitamins makes the body to have high immunity.

Squash also has magnesium and phosphorus which helps to make the bones strong also the teeth will be strong. This prevent unhealthy teeth and bones.

After eating, it is good to brush the

teeth with toothbrush and fluoride

toothpaste this prevent tooth caries

and dental cavity.

Salad is very good for the body. It

makes the vessels of the body young.

It makes the heart to have normal

shape and looks healthy. It prevent

liver diseases. It prevent kidney

diseases. It prevent lungs diseases. It

prevent brain diseases. It makes the

whole body to be young and healthy.

It makes the body to have a lot of

minerals and vitamins that will make

the immunity of the whole body to

be high. It makes the body to fight

against infections. This makes

diseases to be prevented.

Salad assists the leukocytes (white

blood cells) to fight against

infections. Salads makes the bone

marrow to produce blood cells. This

makes anemia to be prevented.

Salad prevent cancer. It makes

mitosis and meiosis to occur

normally in the body, thereby causing growth and development to occur normally in the body.

It is very good to drink enough water to keep the body fit. It is good to so have exercise to keep the body in normal condition.

It is good for parents to let the children know the importance of salad. It's health benefits. And how the information can be known world wide.

It is also good to teach pupils in

school on the nutritional benefits of

salad. Salad makes the body to be

normal.

www.ingramcontent.com/pod-product-compliance
Lightning Source LLC
Chambersburg PA
CBHW031140250726
48655CB00002B/761